HERBAL HAIR OIL

PRODUCTION

Easy Guide To Herbal Hair Oil Production
Full Course On How To Produce Effective Herbal Hair Oil
Be A Formulator Not A Mixer.

All right reserved. No part of this publication may be reproduced, distributed or transmitted in any form or by any means, including photocopying, recording, or other electronic or mechanical methods, without the prior written permission of the publisher, expect in any case of brief questions embodied in critical reviews and certain other noncommercial uses permitted by copyright law

Jessica R. Lampe

DEDICATION

This guide is dedicated to those who love natural hair products and to those who found it difficult to grow their hair and have probably used different hair care products in order to maintain their healthy natural hair but none of them worked..

Jessica R. Lampe

COURSE OUTLINE

TABLE OF CONTENT

Jessica R. Lampe

Jessica R. Lampe

INTRODUCTION

Currently hair care oils are moving from chemical-base ingredients to all natural ingredients, carrier oil and essential oil.

Herbal hair oil hydrates the scalp while also reversing the effect of dry scalp and hair. The most important one is Herbal hair oil supports growth and healthy hair within a short period of time.

Herbal hair oil contains a variety of vital nutrients from herbs, carrier oil and essential oil that help the sebaceous gland operate normally and promote natural hair growth.

Herbal hair oil mainly comprises oil of vegetable extracts in origin as base and blended with suitable herbs that support hair growth and repair.

Sadly, you've been wondering why commercial brands sell herbal hair oil expensive and it comes in small form while some other commercial brands sell herbal hair oil at affordable price and when you receive it, it will not be herbal hair oil and might contain different unnatural material that may cause damage to your hair scalp and hair.

This is the main reason why we create this herbal hair oil recipe that is affordable and can be done at home for personal use or selling purpose.

Jessica R. Lampe

One of the Major hair care treatments is herbal hair oil. This oil will offer benefits of organic oils and natural herbs to the hair and scalp.

Applying herbal hair oil into the hair will enhance the strands' straighten and aid the improvement of the hair.
The moment herbs are infused in oil it supplies benefits that support hair growth, hair repair, prevent hair damages and other hair issues.

THIS BOOK IS ALL ABOUT THE FOLLOWING

How to calculate product formula
How to calculate percentage in gram for your production
Know your hair type and hair porosity for a perfect hair care routine
Benefits of herbal hair oil and why you should use herbal hair oil for your hair care routine
How to properly produce effective herbal hair oil
Perfect ingredients to use for your herbal hair oil production
How to have a healthy, shiny, long hair
How to maintain a good and healthy scalp
This eBook is your resource guide on how to DIY herbal hair oil.

Jessica R. Lampe

CHAPTER 1

HAIR CARE

Hair care in general terms for hygiene involves the hair which grows from the human scalp.

Hair to us as human beings is a fundamental expression of the way we were created. No wonder when the hair is looking at its best, you always feel good and look radiant. No matter how simple it is taking care of hair, you don't want to do it wrongly most times, it is not about how the products are being used, but the type of hair care products been used

According to my research 90% of women are not okay with the way their hair looks and are ready to trade it with anything. Some expect even suggested that apart from face beauty, hair is another reason why most women get a good number of compliments.

Jessica R. Lampe

In the case of Men a d Woman 70% of men are suffering from baldness, alopecia. My recent research alopecia affected and estimated 50 million men and 30 million women in the US in 2023. And estimated future reach in 2025 will be approximately 80 million men and 50 million women.

People are now looking for products that will take care of their hair with fewer chemicals on their hair.

This change in orientation led to the popularity of herbal care treatment and products..

IMPORTANCE OF HAIR CARE

You really don't need to be schooled on how important it is to take good care of your hair. It is your hair that makes you attractive and beautiful as the case may be. After flawless skin, face beauty, your hair plays a vital role in physical appearance. Having healthy hair boosts your confidence as a lady.

Experience has shown that some hair care products can cause dryness and scalp itching because of the harsh chemical ingredients.

With some simple steps, you can reduce damage that those products may want to do your hair:

Jessica R. Lampe

<u>Wash your hair regularly</u>: whenever you wash your hair, you must massage the scalp to keep it clean and healthy. No that a clean scalp makes a healthy hair

<u>Hairstyle</u>: the way you style your hair matters in hair care, making hair that thug and pull your hair will cause you to lose your hair over time.

<u>Choose the appropriate hair care</u>: most of the hair care products out there contain harsh chemicals that will damage hair. So the best advice is to use hair care products that contain natural base ingredients.

<u>Blow-dryer</u>: I truly do not suggest utilizing blow-dryer to dry up your hair since of the warm, you can effortlessly dry with your towel to diminish harm to your scalp.

<u>Break time</u>: it is essential and very important to give your hair a break at times. Don't use any hair care products on it for some time, allow it to be natural.

<u>Trim your hair</u>: if you want your hair to look good and healthy make it a habit to trim it. Growing good healthy hair requires proper time, hair it's just like grass growing, some parts will damage along the growth process. You have to cut it out to allow the good ones to grow properly and healthy.

Jessica R. Lampe

<u>Feed your hair</u>: your hair needs substances like vitamin, protein and mineral-rich food to thrive. Those substances will help the hair to grow and develop.

Last but not the least, also give your hair hot oil treatment if you want it to shine and be less prone to damage.

MOST COMMON HAIR CARE ISSUE

Every woman would want a healthy shiny long and beautiful hair and achieving this feat be a challenge
Having good hair requires time and money and appropriate maintenance. 90% Hair problems can be a product of different types of factors that include environmental, genetic, chemical and mechanical. Here there are several stresses throughout the day, and It can be challenging to bring them back to health and balance.

The Factors Below Are Some Of The Most Common Hair Issues.

OILY AND GREASY HAIR

Human skin is full of pores joined to sebaceous glands that reveal a natural oil known as sebum. It is the function of sebum to keep hair manageable, soft and smooth.

Jessica R. Lampe

Factors that cause oily and greasy hair may be natural causes that include hair type, hormones, genetics and skin condition like eczema and psoriasis.

Other causes that are human made are frequent brushing of hair, frequent shampooing and conditioning of hair or trying your hair too tight.

Another cause that we are not serious about is regular use of hot water on your hair, hot water stimulates the sebaceous glands and makes them produce more sebum.

DANDRUFF

Dandruff can be referred to as a skin condition that mainly affects the scalp. Symptoms include peeling and flaking. Most times individuals thought that this side effect is a sign of destitute cleanliness but numerous reasons contribute to dandruff.

Among other reasons, seborrheic dermatitis can cause several dandruff. This is a situation when the skin is overactive, thereby leading to the scalp being irritated and producing extra skin cells.

When the skin cells die, they will fall off and form what is known as dandruff. Is Wendy skin is too dry, especially during winter also, trigger a red, itchy scalp

SENSITIVE SCALPS

When the scalp is sensitive, it will be feeling itchy and irritated. When the scalp cap is sensitive, it will bring out some conditions such as tightness, itchiness, and there will be pain at the roots. The imbalance of sebum secretion that leads to irritation can be one of the sources of scalp sensitively. Pollution of coast hair can also be one of the causes as it will create a dull film on the hair and create free medicals.

COLOR AND BLEACH DAMAGE HAIR

Chemicals are exposed to hair when you dye. These harsh chemicals can lead to hair damage. Whenever the hair is exposed to harsh chemicals, the hair becomes very porous and filled with small holes due to color.
Bleaching of hair raises its outer cuticle for the bleaching agent to penetrate. When repeated bleaching of the hair we build the cuticle scale, thereby allowing it to lose moisture. Bleaching will lead to hair being broken and having split ends.

HEAT DAMAGE HAIR

Styling of straight, wave or curly hair requires hot tools, a good way to make your hair look nice, the problems come when you overuse or are incorrectly used. Heat damage may help pin in one simple curl or swipe when overexposed to them.

HAIR LOSS

Hair loss leads to low self-esteem. Hair loss occurs when the androgen hormones in the body that shrink hair follicles are not growing again. Is certainly not the only reason for hair loss, and it may be due to alopecia areata and autoimmune situations where an immune system attacks the hair follicle.
It may also be a result of hormonal imbalance that occurs during pregnancy. Hair loss can sometimes be a result of medical treatment and sickness.
Another factor is when the body has gone through sudden stress which will lead to hair loss.

DRY HAIR

When hair is finding it challenging to return the moisture, if you need to dry hair. Dry hair is a condition when the hair will be less shiny, appearing dull and lifeless. It is a sign of unhealthy hair, and those different kinds of factors that include environmental condition, hair condition and exposure to harsh products are part of what may have caused it.
Dry climates, frequent swimming in salty or chlorinated water, and much exposure to wind or sun, is part of the environmental factors that affect hair. Others are exposure to harsh chemicals, frequent washing of hair, dying of hair, and frequent use of blow dryer straightener and curling iron.

Jessica R. Lampe

HAIR POROSITY

Hair porosity can be defined as the ability of your hair to soak up and hold moisture and products. There are three levels of porosity which include low porosity, medium porosity and high porosity.

<u>LOW POROSITY</u>: low porosity refers to human hair that does not absorb water or products easily. Your hair may have low porosity if it takes a long time to absorb water. If the products you use to take care of your hair tend to remain on the surface instead of being absorbed your hair is Low porosity.
<u>MEDIUM POROSITY</u>: medium porosity is human hair that absorbs water slowly, it's halfway open that moisture can reach inside the hair shaft.

<u>HIGH POROSITY</u>: high porosity is a human hair that quickly absorbs and loses moisture due to gaps and holes in the cuticle layer. This can lead to a lot of issues such as weak strands, breakage, split ends.

Understanding your hair porosity you can solve 30% of your hair problems, knowing products that can be good for your hair and how to use them

<u>HOW YO CHECK HAIR POROSITY</u>: first is a glass of water test. Simply take a clean strand of hair and put it in a glass of water.
If the hair strand floats at the top your hair is low porosity.
If the hair strand sinks slowly and settles in the middle your hair is medium porosity.

Jessica R. Lampe

If the hair strand sinks straight to the bottom of the water your hair is a high porosity. This is a proper way which you can check your hair porosity.

Above listed are only equipment you need to buy before production. Note if you are Open For Business kindly get those items in a digger form of it.

HOW TO CLEAN AND STORE YOUR EQUIPMENT AFTER PRODUCTION

Easy guide on how you properly store your equipment after production.

Hygiene is very necessary when producing anything being used by humans, production equipment is meant to be clean before production in order not to add bacteria to the products.

STEP BY STEP GUIDE

You should follow the manufacturer's instructions in cleaning any electronic equipment. Other equipment that is not electronic here is the proper way which you can clean them after production.

Step 1: add all your equipment in a transparent plastic bowl add warm water and detergent than wash properly

Jessica R. Lampe

Step 2: rinse with clean water, it must be utilized to remove all traces and detergent.
Step 3: Dry with a clean soft cloth before allowing it to dry properly

Step4: Put in a dry plastic container and tightly close it for next time use.

Jessica R. Lampe

CHAPTER 4

WHAT IS HERB

Herbs generally refer to the leafy green or flowering parts of a plant (either fresh or dried) that are useful for medicinal, aromatic and savory properties.

BENEFIT OF HEEBS

Herbs have a lot of benefits to the human body. Consuming herbs may help to prevent and manage heart disease, cancer, diabetes, hair, brain, skin etc..

WAY TO PREPARE HERBS

We have different ways in which you can prepare herbs. The preparation of herbs depends on the purpose of what you want to use it for. We will be looking into oil infusion because this book is all about herbal hair oil which we will focus on.

OIL INFUSION: Oil infusion is the combination of different herbs and oil in order to form a product. Recommending using grinded dry herbs for perfect results.

Jessica R. Lampe

Infusion Process Has Two Methods

Method 1: Infusing herbs in oil with the method of double boiling in order to infuse fast this process can be done if you are urgently using the product and to fasting the infusion process.

Method 2: Infusing herbs in oil usually takes a long time. If you're not using the double boiling method, you can infuse herbs in oil for 4 weeks. 4 weeks allow the herbs to infuse properly in the oil without double boiling.

WHAT IS CARRIER OIL

Carrier Oils are Vegetable oils that are obtained from the fatty parts of plants—typically the seeds, kernels, or nuts.

There Are Variety Of Of Carrier Oils, Including

Argan, Olive, Jojoba, Coconut, and many more. In order to apply concentrated essential oils to the skin without risking negative reactions, carrier oils dilute the oils.

FEW BENEFITS OF CARRIER OILS

There are numerous health benefits of carrier oil for humans; I'll list a few here. Carrier oils moisturize and soften skin, and even help reduce inflammation from skin disorders like eczema, hydrate hair. It's simple to make your own hair and skin care products without the use of harmful chemicals by blending carrier oils and essential oils.

Jessica R. Lampe

ESSENTIAL OILS

Essential oils reduce tension, cure fungus infections, have a pleasant scent, and promote restful sleep. These are concentrated plant extracts. Plant "essence" can be transformed into a liquid form for a variety of therapeutic and recreational purposes using a process known as distillation. Selection of essential oils is extensive. There are a variety of essential oils, such as tea tree oil, orange oil, rosemary oil etc..

Jessica R. Lampe

CHAPTER 5

FORMULATION

A formulation is a mixture of ingredients prepared in a certain way and used for a specific purpose.

CREATING A FORMULATION.

When Creating A Formulation, it is essential you write it down first, get a sheet of paper and write out your formula; I understand it is very tempting to want to rush off to start, but you have to take this very slowly and do it step by step.

•STEP 1- Get a sheet of paper or formulation book.

•STEP 2- Write out the ingredients you intend using (Start in a small batch to avoid waste of ingredients if you're selling)

•STEP 3- Calculate your percentage and convert them to grams.Doing this will enable you to recreate your products over and over again.

•STEP 4- Ensure that your products retain the same mixture,scent. By doing this, people will mark you out as a professional hair care formulator, not a mixer.

Jessica R. Lampe

*HOW TO CALCULATE FORMULAS

In this material, I would be teaching you how to calculate your recipes in percentage and convert them into grams. You need to be able to turn your recipe's percentage into a gram formula for your records, so that once you are in business, you can make this product over and over at any size, without being different each time you produce it. It is always best to record all your formulas as percentage formulas and then work out the weight-based formula when you head into the lab to cook up a batch of a product, so just in case, you have been working in weight so far,this is the best chance for you to learn how to turn your current formulas in percentages and easily make a large batch as you wish.

WAYS TO CALCULATE YOUR RECIPES

(CONVERTING PERCENTAGE TO GRAMS)

Firstly you will need to first decide on your batch size (how much products you want to make) you can choose any amount in grams or ml (grams and ml are the same thing in skincare/haircare)
Then turn your percentage based formula into weight
based measurement depending on the batch size.

The calculation you need

Percentage of the ingredients(divided by) 100
(multiply by) batch size = weight of the ingredients

Jessica R. Lampe

FOR EXAMPLE

We are using this scrub recipe as a case study. We are producing 100g of scrub. The 100g is our batch size

Almond oil - Foundation   35%
Jojoba oil   - Foundation   15%

Sugar - Functional   37%
Green tea - Botanical   5%
Coffee powder - Botanical   5%
Vitamin E - Antioxidant   1%
Geranium - Essential oil   1%
Germall plus - Preservative   1%

THE CALCULATION WILL BE

1. Almond oil 35% (don't forget anything in % is over 100) It will be 35/100 multiply by100= 35g

2. Jojoba oil 15%   15/100 multiply 100=15g

3.Sugar 37%   37/100 multiply by 100=37g

4.Green tea 5%   5/100 multiply by 100=5g

5.Coffee powder 5%   5/100 multiply by 100 =5g

6.Vitamin E 1%   1/100 multiply by 100= 1g

Jessica R. Lampe

7.Geranium 1%   1/100 multiply by 100= 1g
8.Germall plus 1%   1/100 multiply by 100= 1g

TOTAL OF ALL THE INGREDIENTS IN GRAMS=100g

Check your calculation afterward as it should always add up to 100g, the total gram size of what you intend to make.

Now you know the method for calculating percentages in formulas from an existing recipe. It is vital to keep all your records as percentage formulas; that way, you will be able to keep reproducing those products over and over, and they will always be the same. No matter what size you make it, it doesn't matter if you make 5,000 gram size the result will be the same.
Keep practicing and recreate % for other recipes.

FORMULATION CHALLENGES

Formulation challenges, ranging from regulations, product safety,aesthetics and so on.To be a successful formulator,one must toggle many priorities with limited resources.

Every Ingredient Should Have a Function.

A Formulator should understand the structure-property relationship and the role of each raw material in a formula.Raw materials are tools for creating formulation options and contributing to sensory,stability and efficaciousness of the formulation.

Jessica R. Lampe

There are many cosmetic ingredients with multiple functions,providing benefits that meet consumer demands.By understanding the ingredient function and interactions in the complex composition,A formulator can develop better formulation strategies.

At times, a formulator would be asked to "tweak" an existing formulation in order to replace an ingredient in response to a customer's demand or brand need.

NOTE; Simply piling lot of ingredients into a formula does not always provide a solution to the problem.In fact, it can backfire and create instability,or other unwanted issues that would lead to trouble and requires a formulator dealing with fixing a failed recipe which automatically can lead to waste of money,time and resources.

It is important to be familiar with the latest raw material technology and formulation.
One way to quickly become familiar with formulation is understanding raw materials used in a formula by studying its full ingredient list, reading competitor's list and publications,and last but not least create,revise and test until the desired aesthetics you wish are obtained.

A cosmetic formulator could be asked to "reformulate" an existing product formulation.This approach can save time and resources on efficacy and safety testing,strategy pertains to raw material replacement in a formula,take time to read

Jessica R. Lampe

ingredients substitution and usage of the new ingredients,if old ingredients in formula are not available in the market i.e., replacing raw materials based on how they function in the formulation.if you wish to change an ingredient because it's not available in the market to purchase.

<u>WHAT IS PRODUCTION</u>

Production is simply the process of making or manufacturing goods and products from raw materials or components.

CHAPTER 6

HERBAL HAIR OIL

Herbal hair oil is the combination of herbs, carrier oils and essential oils to form a hair oil.

HERBS

•Red Ginseng Root Extract Powder
•Basil powder
•Ginkgo Biloba Powder
•Nettle Powder
•Cloves
•Rose Petals
•Hibiscus Flower
•Rosemary leaves
•Ashwagandha Powder
•Brahmi Powder
•Neem Powder
•Shikakai Powder
•Amla Powder
•Henna Powder
•Moringa Powder
•Fennel seed

•Black Seed
•Fenugreek Powder
•Bhringraj powder
•Chebe powder

CARRIER OILS

•Olive Oil
•Argan Oil
•Coconut Oil
•Jamaican Black Castor oil
•Batana oil

ESSENTIAL OIL

•Lavender oil

How To Calculate Herbal Hair Oil; In the production of herbal hair oil, olive oil is the Foundation (Base) of the production in which the percentage will be higher than other oils.

Other oils are the additional oils that boost the effect of the products while herbs are the actives that supply effects to the oil which will be removed after infusion.

Jessica R. Lampe

The way you calculate your hair Scrub, hair cream or anything that has no herbs in it that only contains butters and oil is different from the way you calculate hair oils or anything that has herbs to infuse in it. You're to Calculate herbs and oil differently and to give you 100% of what you want to produce.

We are producing 1000 Grams of herbal hair oil (1000g is 1 liter)

You are to calculate the oil percentage to 100% and calculate the herbs to 100%

Oil calculation should give you 100% of what you intend to produce

herbs should also give you 100% of what you intend to produce

Herbal Hair Oil Calculation

OIL PERCENTAGE
•Olive Oil 60%
•Argan Oil 10%
•Coconut Oil 10 %
•Jamaican Black Castor oil 5%
•Lavender oil 10%
•Batana oil 5%

Total 100%

HERBS PERCENTAGE

•Red Ginseng Root Extract Powder 20%
•Basil powder 10%
•Ginkgo Biloba Powder   5%
•Nettle Powder 5%
•Cloves 4%
•Rose Petals   3%
•Hibiscus Flower 3%
•Rosemary leaves 3%
•Ashwagandha Powder 7%
•Brahmi Powder 3%
•Neem Powder 3%
•Shikakai Powder 3%
•Amla Powder 5%
•Henna Powder 3%
•Moringa Powder 4%
•Fennel seed 5%
•Black Seed 5%
•Fenugreek Powder 2%
•Bhringraj powder 5%
•Chebe powder 2%

Total 100%

TAKE NOTES

Jessica R. Lampe

I recommend you add extra 500ml of your base oil when producing because after infusion and straining the oil from the herbs there will be little oil that is stuck in the herbs and which will reduce the size of what you intend to achieve but adding 500 grams to your production gives you extra grams. Even if some oil is stuck in the herbs you will achieve the size you intend to produce with a little leftover oil.

<u>LET'S QUICKLY GO OF TO PRODUCTION STEPS</u>

HOW TO PRODUCE HERBAL HAIR OIL

STEP 1: In a plastic or stainless container, add in your base Oil (Olive oil) with the extra 500 grams
STEP 2: Add herbs to the base, and stir properly
STEP 3: Allow the herbs to infuse for 4 weeks

4 weeks allow the seeds and herbs to properly infuse in the oil, stir the mixture every 5 days for proper infusion.

STEP 4: After the infusion state, strain the oil from the herbs
STEP 5: Add the carrier oils and essential oil to the mixture and stir properly, allow to sit for 1 hour. It's ready to use

This oil lasts more than 6 months when you properly store it.

SECOND METHOD WHICH YOU CAN PRODUCE HAIR OIL IN 7 DAYS

Jessica R. Lampe

STEP 1: in a plastic or stainless container add in your base oil (Olive oil) with the extra 500 grams

STEP 2: Add the herbs to the base and stir properly to mix together

STEP 3: Allow the herbs to infuse for 7 days

STEP 4: As we are working on 7 days infusion we will add a double boiling method to fasten the infusion process.

DOUBLE BOILING is the method which you can place a pot of water in a low heat, add in the mixture in a clean stainless bowl and place on top of the water, allow to double boil for 20 to 30 minutes or when you started perceiving the smell of the oil, turn off the heater and allow the mixture to cool down.

STEP 5: Add the carrier oils and essential oil to the mixture and stir properly, allow to sit for 1 hour. It's ready to use

Properly package your oil in a big container or jar and store in a clean dry place.

Jessica R. Lampe

USAGE

Below are listed usage options for your hair type carefully read the usage option in order to use herbal hair oil properly. Like I said you should get a 100 ml dropper bottle or small bottle to retail the oil for easy to apply.

If it is a dropper bottle don't allow the mouth of the dropper to touch your scalp or skin, raise the dropper a little bit and drop on your scalp then massage properly for a safety product.

LOW POROSITY HAIR As a low porosity hair you are to apply herbal hair oil morning and night 5 times in a week. add a few drops of hair oil direct your scalp and massage properly. *Constant use to achieve better results.*

When you achieve the length you want for your hair you can easily apply the hair oil two times in a week to retain the moisture and health.

MEDIUM POROSITY HAIR As a medium porosity hair, you are to apply herbal hair oil every night and cover your hair before you go to bed. Apply herbal hair oil 4 times in a week *Constant use to achieve better results.*

When you achieve the results you want for your hair you can apply the oil two times in a week to retain the moisture and health.

Jessica R. Lampe

HIGH POROSITY HAIR As a high porosity hair, you are to apply herbal hair oil morning and night everyday, add a few drops directly to your hair scalp and massage.
Constant use to achieve better results.

When you achieve the results you want for your hair you can apply the oil two times in a week to retain the moisture and health.

HOT OILS SCALP TREATMENT

- Heat the oil in a pot
- Separate your hair into 4 to 6 sections
- Add few drops to you scalp
- Message the oil into your roots and drag to the end of your hair
- Cover your hair with a shower cap for 30 minutes
- Shampoo your hair

BENEFITS OF HERBAL HAIR OIL

1: Herbal hair oil hydrates and smoothing the hair and scalp, treats dandruff and prevents shedding and hair Fall.

2: Herbal hair oil repair any scalp and hair issue like alopecia, baldness, hair fall, hair shedding, breakage, thin hair, edges repair etc and also prevent scalp issues

Jessica R. Lampe

3: Adding herbal hair oil to your hair care routine, it fasting the growth process, if your current products is not effective you can easily include this herbal hair oil to your hair care routine it will fasting the growth process and allow other products to penetrate in your scalp

4: Herbal hair oil helps in blood circulation to the scalp and maintain scalp health for health and long hair

5: with the moisturizing agent in our herbal hair oil, Herbal hair oil supply nutrients to the scalp, improve moisture retention in the strands and moisturize the hair

6: herbal hair oil nourish hair follicles, strengthen hair strands and improve the overall health of your hair

7: Herbal hair oil stimulate hair follicles and promote stronger, healthier and growth of the roots

8: Herbal hair oil work as antifungal property and help combat dandruff and promote a healthy scalp

9: Herbal hair oil contains rich vitamins and regrows hair.

10: Herbal hair oil works for all kinds of hair type, texture and porosity. You don't need to worry about your hair type when using this herbal hair oil, properly go through the usage option of your hair type.

Jessica R. Lampe

CONCLUSION

As we come to the conclusion of herbal hair oil production, how you can properly formulate and produce herbal hair oil.

As a beginner in formulator, for you not to waste your resources, start producing in small batches for training purposes.

Rushing to produce a bigger quantity might result in waste of resources or mistakes in production if you intend to get this book for a business purpose.

As you are still a beginner you have to follow the steps, don't skip any part in order to start formulating, go through the steps, go through the calculation, train yourself three times if you get the same results you can produce any batch you want for your oil.

And follow the usage option for your hair type. Also check your hair type before using this oil to achieve better results.

Jessica R. Lampe